Make-Up Face Sheet
Portfolio

by Andreea Iosif

This portfolio belongs to: ....

Face Sheet

Name:...Date:...........................Client Ref:..

SKIN TONES
FOUNDATION & CONCEALER

- Light
- Medium
- Dark

SKIN ONDITIONS

- Young
- Mature

EYES

MAKE-UP CONTEXTS

- Day
- Evening
- Bridal

TECHNIQUES

- Correction - Warming
- Correction - Cooling
- Concealing
- Bronzing
- Highlighting
- Shading
- Strip Lashes
- Individual Lashes

CHEEKS

FASHION STYLE

LIPS

PERIOD STYLE

ADDITIONAL TECHNIQUES

Note:

Is this client contraindicated? ☐ YES ☐ NO

This is evidence of:

☐ Class Work ☐ Home Work ☐ Internal Evaluation ☐ External Examination

CONTRA-ACTIONS	
AFTERCARE ADVICE	
HOME CARE ADVICE	
CLIENT/ MODEL SIGNATURE	TEACHER/ EXAMINER SIGNATURE

Face Sheet

Name:...............................Date:..........................Client Ref:...

SKIN TONES	FOUNDATION & CONCEALER
Light
Medium
Dark

SKIN ONDITIONS
Young
Mature

EYES

MAKE-UP CONTEXTS
Day
Evening
Bridal

TECHNIQUES
Correction - Warming
Correction - Cooling
Concealing
Bronzing
Highlighting
Shading
Strip Lashes
Individual Lashes

CHEEKS

FASHION STYLE

LIPS

PERIOD STYLE

ADDITIONAL TECHNIQUES

Note:

Is this client contraindicated? ☐ YES ☐ NO

This is evidence of:

☐ Class Work ☐ Home Work ☐ Internal Evaluation ☐ External Examination

CONTRA-ACTIONS	
AFTERCARE ADVICE	
HOME CARE ADVICE	
CLIENT/ MODEL SIGNATURE	TEACHER/ EXAMINER SIGNATURE

Face Sheet

Name:.................................Date:...........................Client Ref:...

SKIN TONES

Light
Medium
Dark

SKIN ONDITIONS

Young
Mature

MAKE-UP CONTEXTS

Day
Evening
Bridal

TECHNIQUES

Correction - Warming
Correction - Cooling
Concealing
Bronzing
Highlighting
Shading
Strip Lashes
Individual Lashes

FASHION STYLE

PERIOD STYLE

ADDITIONAL TECHNIQUES

FOUNDATION & CONCEALER

EYES

CHEEKS

LIPS

Note:

Is this client contraindicated? ☐ YES ☐ NO

This is evidence of:

☐ Class Work ☐ Home Work ☐ Internal Evaluation ☐ External Examination

CONTRA-ACTIONS	
AFTERCARE ADVICE	
HOME CARE ADVICE	
CLIENT/ MODEL SIGNATURE	TEACHER/ EXAMINER SIGNATURE

Face Sheet

Name:.............................Date:............................Client Ref:......................................

SKIN TONES
Light
Medium
Dark

SKIN ONDITIONS
Young
Mature

MAKE-UP CONTEXTS
Day
Evening
Bridal

TECHNIQUES
Correction - Warming
Correction - Cooling
Concealing
Bronzing
Highlighting
Shading
Strip Lashes
Individual Lashes

FASHION STYLE

PERIOD STYLE

ADDITIONAL TECHNIQUES

FOUNDATION & CONCEALER

EYES

CHEEKS

LIPS

Note:

Is this client contraindicated? ☐ YES   ☐ NO

This is evidence of:

☐ Class Work   ☐ Home Work   ☐ Internal Evaluation   ☐ External Examination

CONTRA-ACTIONS	
AFTERCARE ADVICE	
HOME CARE ADVICE	
CLIENT/ MODEL SIGNATURE	TEACHER/ EXAMINER SIGNATURE

Face Sheet

Name:................................. Date:........................... Client Ref:...........................

SKIN TONES	FOUNDATION & CONCEALER

SKIN TONES
Light
Medium
Dark

SKIN ONDITIONS
Young
Mature

EYES

MAKE-UP CONTEXTS
Day
Evening
Bridal

TECHNIQUES
Correction - Warming
Correction - Cooling
Concealing
Bronzing
Highlighting
Shading
Strip Lashes
Individual Lashes

CHEEKS

FASHION STYLE

LIPS

PERIOD STYLE

ADDITIONAL TECHNIQUES

Note:

Is this client contraindicated? ☐ YES   ☐ NO

This is evidence of:

☐ Class Work   ☐ Home Work   ☐ Internal Evaluation   ☐ External Examination

CONTRA-ACTIONS	
AFTERCARE ADVICE	
HOME CARE ADVICE	
CLIENT/ MODEL SIGNATURE	TEACHER/ EXAMINER SIGNATURE

Face Sheet

Name:................................Date:............................Client Ref:...................................

SKIN TONES	FOUNDATION & CONCEALER
Light	☐
Medium	☐
Dark	☐

SKIN ONDITIONS	
Young	☐
Mature	EYES

MAKE-UP CONTEXTS	
Day	☐
Evening	☐
Bridal	☐

TECHNIQUES	
Correction - Warming	☐
Correction - Cooling	☐
Concealing	☐
Bronzing	CHEEKS
Highlighting	☐
Shading	☐
Strip Lashes	☐
Individual Lashes	☐

FASHION STYLE	LIPS
	☐

PERIOD STYLE	
	☐
	☐

ADDITIONAL TECHNIQUES	

Note:

Is this client contraindicated? ☐ YES ☐ NO

This is evidence of:

☐ Class Work ☐ Home Work ☐ Internal Evaluation ☐ External Examination

CONTRA-ACTIONS	
AFTERCARE ADVICE	
HOME CARE ADVICE	
CLIENT/ MODEL SIGNATURE	TEACHER/ EXAMINER SIGNATURE

Face Sheet

Name:................................ Date:........................ Client Ref:.....................................

SKIN TONES	
Light	
Medium	
Dark	

FOUNDATION & CONCEALER

SKIN ONDITIONS	
Young	
Mature	

EYES

MAKE-UP CONTEXTS	
Day	
Evening	
Bridal	

TECHNIQUES	
Correction - Warming	
Correction - Cooling	
Concealing	
Bronzing	
Highlighting	
Shading	
Strip Lashes	
Individual Lashes	

CHEEKS

FASHION STYLE

LIPS

PERIOD STYLE

ADDITIONAL TECHNIQUES

Note:

Is this client contraindicated? ☐ YES ☐ NO

This is evidence of:

☐ Class Work ☐ Home Work ☐ Internal Evaluation ☐ External Examination

CONTRA-ACTIONS
AFTERCARE ADVICE
HOME CARE ADVICE

CLIENT/ MODEL SIGNATURE	TEACHER/ EXAMINER SIGNATURE

Face Sheet

Name:.............................Date:..........................Client Ref:...............................

SKIN TONES	FOUNDATION & CONCEALER

SKIN TONES
- Light
- Medium
- Dark

SKIN ONDITIONS
- Young
- Mature

MAKE-UP CONTEXTS
- Day
- Evening
- Bridal

TECHNIQUES
- Correction - Warming
- Correction - Cooling
- Concealing
- Bronzing
- Highlighting
- Shading
- Strip Lashes
- Individual Lashes

FASHION STYLE

PERIOD STYLE

ADDITIONAL TECHNIQUES

EYES

CHEEKS

LIPS

Note:

Is this client contraindicated? ☐ YES ☐ NO

This is evidence of:

☐ Class Work ☐ Home Work ☐ Internal Evaluation ☐ External Examination

CONTRA-ACTIONS	
AFTERCARE ADVICE	
HOME CARE ADVICE	
CLIENT/ MODEL SIGNATURE	TEACHER/ EXAMINER SIGNATURE

Face Sheet

Name:................................Date:..........................Client Ref:..............................

SKIN TONES	FOUNDATION & CONCEALER
Light	
Medium	
Dark	

SKIN ONDITIONS	
Young	
Mature	EYES

MAKE-UP CONTEXTS	
Day	
Evening	
Bridal	

TECHNIQUES	
Correction - Warming	
Correction - Cooling	
Concealing	
Bronzing	CHEEKS
Highlighting	
Shading	
Strip Lashes	
Individual Lashes	

FASHION STYLE	LIPS

PERIOD STYLE	

ADDITIONAL TECHNIQUES

Note:

Is this client contraindicated? ☐ YES ☐ NO

This is evidence of:

☐ Class Work ☐ Home Work ☐ Internal Evaluation ☐ External Examination

CONTRA-ACTIONS	
AFTERCARE ADVICE	
HOME CARE ADVICE	
CLIENT/ MODEL SIGNATURE	TEACHER/ EXAMINER SIGNATURE

Face Sheet

Name:............................Date:........................Client Ref:...................................

SKIN TONES
Light
Medium
Dark

SKIN ONDITIONS
Young
Mature

MAKE-UP CONTEXTS
Day
Evening
Bridal

TECHNIQUES
Correction - Warming
Correction - Cooling
Concealing
Bronzing
Highlighting
Shading
Strip Lashes
Individual Lashes

FASHION STYLE

PERIOD STYLE

ADDITIONAL TECHNIQUES

FOUNDATION & CONCEALER

EYES

CHEEKS

LIPS

Note:

Is this client contraindicated?   ☐ YES   ☐ NO

This is evidence of:

☐ Class Work   ☐ Home Work   ☐ Internal Evaluation   ☐ External Examination

CONTRA-ACTIONS	
AFTERCARE ADVICE	
HOME CARE ADVICE	
CLIENT/ MODEL SIGNATURE	TEACHER/ EXAMINER SIGNATURE

Face Sheet

Name:..Date:...........................Client Ref:..

SKIN TONES

Light

Medium

Dark

SKIN ONDITIONS

Young

Mature

MAKE-UP CONTEXTS

Day

Evening

Bridal

TECHNIQUES

Correction - Warming

Correction - Cooling

Concealing

Bronzing

Highlighting

Shading

Strip Lashes

Individual Lashes

FASHION STYLE

PERIOD STYLE

ADDITIONAL TECHNIQUES

FOUNDATION & CONCEALER

EYES

CHEEKS

LIPS

Note:

Is this client contraindicated? ☐ YES ☐ NO

This is evidence of:

☐ Class Work ☐ Home Work ☐ Internal Evaluation ☐ External Examination

CONTRA-ACTIONS	
AFTERCARE ADVICE	
HOME CARE ADVICE	
CLIENT/ MODEL SIGNATURE	TEACHER/ EXAMINER SIGNATURE

Face Sheet

Name:.........................Date:.........................Client Ref:.........................

SKIN TONES
Light
Medium
Dark

SKIN ONDITIONS
Young
Mature

MAKE-UP CONTEXTS
Day
Evening
Bridal

TECHNIQUES
Correction - Warming
Correction - Cooling
Concealing
Bronzing
Highlighting
Shading
Strip Lashes
Individual Lashes

FASHION STYLE

PERIOD STYLE

ADDITIONAL TECHNIQUES

FOUNDATION & CONCEALER

EYES

CHEEKS

LIPS

Note:

Is this client contraindicated? ☐ YES ☐ NO

This is evidence of:

☐ Class Work   ☐ Home Work   ☐ Internal Evaluation   ☐ External Examination

CONTRA-ACTIONS	
AFTERCARE ADVICE	
HOME CARE ADVICE	
CLIENT/ MODEL SIGNATURE	TEACHER/ EXAMINER SIGNATURE

Face Sheet

Name:...........................Date:..........................Client Ref:...

SKIN TONES	FOUNDATION & CONCEALER
Light	☐
Medium	☐
Dark	☐

SKIN ONDITIONS	
Young	☐
Mature	☐

EYES

MAKE-UP CONTEXTS	
Day	☐
Evening	☐
Bridal	☐

TECHNIQUES	
Correction - Warming	☐
Correction - Cooling	☐
Concealing	☐
Bronzing	☐
Highlighting	
Shading	☐
Strip Lashes	☐
Individual Lashes	☐

CHEEKS

FASHION STYLE
☐

LIPS

PERIOD STYLE
☐

ADDITIONAL TECHNIQUES

Note:

Is this client contraindicated? ☐ YES ☐ NO

This is evidence of:

☐ Class Work ☐ Home Work ☐ Internal Evaluation ☐ External Examination

CONTRA-ACTIONS	
AFTERCARE ADVICE	
HOME CARE ADVICE	
CLIENT/ MODEL SIGNATURE	TEACHER/ EXAMINER SIGNATURE

Face Sheet

Name:...........................Date:...........................Client Ref:...........................

FOUNDATION & CONCEALER

SKIN TONES
- Light
- Medium
- Dark

SKIN ONDITIONS
- Young
- Mature

EYES

MAKE-UP CONTEXTS
- Day
- Evening
- Bridal

TECHNIQUES
- Correction - Warming
- Correction - Cooling
- Concealing
- Bronzing
- Highlighting
- Shading
- Strip Lashes
- Individual Lashes

CHEEKS

FASHION STYLE

LIPS

PERIOD STYLE

ADDITIONAL TECHNIQUES

Note:

Is this client contraindicated? ☐ YES ☐ NO

This is evidence of:

☐ Class Work ☐ Home Work ☐ Internal Evaluation ☐ External Examination

CONTRA-ACTIONS
AFTERCARE ADVICE
HOME CARE ADVICE

CLIENT/ MODEL SIGNATURE	TEACHER/ EXAMINER SIGNATURE

Face Sheet

Name:....................................Date:...........................Client Ref:...

SKIN TONES

Light	
Medium	
Dark	

SKIN ONDITIONS

Young	
Mature	

MAKE-UP CONTEXTS

Day	
Evening	
Bridal	

TECHNIQUES

Correction - Warming	
Correction - Cooling	
Concealing	
Bronzing	
Highlighting	
Shading	
Strip Lashes	
Individual Lashes	

FASHION STYLE

PERIOD STYLE

ADDITIONAL TECHNIQUES

FOUNDATION & CONCEALER

EYES

CHEEKS

LIPS

Note:

Is this client contraindicated?   ☐ YES   ☐ NO

This is evidence of:

☐ Class Work   ☐ Home Work   ☐ Internal Evaluation   ☐ External Examination

CONTRA-ACTIONS	
AFTERCARE ADVICE	
HOME CARE ADVICE	
CLIENT/ MODEL SIGNATURE	TEACHER/ EXAMINER SIGNATURE

Face Sheet

Name:................................Date:............................Client Ref:.....................................

SKIN TONES	FOUNDATION & CONCEALER
Light	☐
Medium	☐
Dark	☐

SKIN ONDITIONS	
Young	☐
Mature	EYES

MAKE-UP CONTEXTS	
Day	☐
Evening	☐
Bridal	☐

TECHNIQUES	
Correction - Warming	☐
Correction - Cooling	☐
Concealing	☐
Bronzing	CHEEKS
Highlighting	☐
Shading	☐
Strip Lashes	☐
Individual Lashes	☐

FASHION STYLE	LIPS
	☐

PERIOD STYLE	
	☐
	☐

ADDITIONAL TECHNIQUES

Note:

Is this client contraindicated?   ☐ YES   ☐ NO

This is evidence of:

☐ Class Work   ☐ Home Work   ☐ Internal Evaluation   ☐ External Examination

CONTRA-ACTIONS	
AFTERCARE ADVICE	
HOME CARE ADVICE	
CLIENT/ MODEL SIGNATURE	TEACHER/ EXAMINER SIGNATURE

Face Sheet

Name:................................ Date:......................... Client Ref:..................................

SKIN TONES	FOUNDATION & CONCEALER
Light	☐
Medium	☐
Dark	☐

SKIN ONDITIONS

Young	☐
Mature	EYES

MAKE-UP CONTEXTS

Day	☐
Evening	☐
Bridal	☐

TECHNIQUES

Correction - Warming	☐
Correction - Cooling	☐
Concealing	☐
Bronzing	CHEEKS
Highlighting	☐
Shading	☐
Strip Lashes	☐
Individual Lashes	☐

FASHION STYLE

LIPS ☐

PERIOD STYLE

☐
☐

ADDITIONAL TECHNIQUES

Note:

Is this client contraindicated?   ☐ YES   ☐ NO

This is evidence of:

☐ Class Work   ☐ Home Work   ☐ Internal Evaluation   ☐ External Examination

CONTRA-ACTIONS	
AFTERCARE ADVICE	
HOME CARE ADVICE	
CLIENT/ MODEL SIGNATURE	TEACHER/ EXAMINER SIGNATURE

Face Sheet

Name:................................Date:...........................Client Ref:.................................

SKIN TONES
Light
Medium
Dark

SKIN ONDITIONS
Young
Mature

MAKE-UP CONTEXTS
Day
Evening
Bridal

TECHNIQUES
Correction - Warming
Correction - Cooling
Concealing
Bronzing
Highlighting
Shading
Strip Lashes
Individual Lashes

FASHION STYLE

PERIOD STYLE

ADDITIONAL TECHNIQUES

FOUNDATION & CONCEALER

EYES

CHEEKS

LIPS

Note:

Is this client contraindicated? ☐ YES ☐ NO

This is evidence of:

☐ Class Work ☐ Home Work ☐ Internal Evaluation ☐ External Examination

CONTRA-ACTIONS	
AFTERCARE ADVICE	
HOME CARE ADVICE	
CLIENT/ MODEL SIGNATURE	TEACHER/ EXAMINER SIGNATURE

Face Sheet

Name:............................... Date:............................... Client Ref:..

SKIN TONES	FOUNDATION & CONCEALER
Light	☐
Medium	☐
Dark	☐

SKIN ONDITIONS	
Young	☐
Mature	☐
	EYES

MAKE-UP CONTEXTS	
Day	☐
Evening	☐
Bridal	☐

TECHNIQUES	
Correction - Warming	☐
Correction - Cooling	☐
Concealing	☐
Bronzing	CHEEKS
Highlighting	
Shading	☐
Strip Lashes	☐
Individual Lashes	☐

FASHION STYLE	LIPS
	☐

PERIOD STYLE	
	☐

ADDITIONAL TECHNIQUES

Note:

Is this client contraindicated?   ☐ YES   ☐ NO

This is evidence of:

☐ Class Work   ☐ Home Work   ☐ Internal Evaluation   ☐ External Examination

CONTRA-ACTIONS	
AFTERCARE ADVICE	
HOME CARE ADVICE	
CLIENT/ MODEL SIGNATURE	TEACHER/ EXAMINER SIGNATURE

Face Sheet

Name:.......................... Date:...................... Client Ref:.................................

SKIN TONES	FOUNDATION & CONCEALER

SKIN TONES
- Light ☐
- Medium ☐
- Dark ☐

SKIN ONDITIONS
- Young ☐
- Mature ☐

EYES

MAKE-UP CONTEXTS
- Day ☐
- Evening ☐
- Bridal ☐

TECHNIQUES
- Correction - Warming ☐
- Correction - Cooling ☐
- Concealing ☐
- Bronzing ☐

CHEEKS

- Highlighting ☐
- Shading ☐
- Strip Lashes ☐
- Individual Lashes ☐

FASHION STYLE
☐

LIPS

PERIOD STYLE
☐
☐

ADDITIONAL TECHNIQUES

Note:

Is this client contraindicated? ☐ YES ☐ NO

This is evidence of:

☐ Class Work ☐ Home Work ☐ Internal Evaluation ☐ External Examination

CONTRA-ACTIONS	
AFTERCARE ADVICE	
HOME CARE ADVICE	
CLIENT/ MODEL SIGNATURE	TEACHER/ EXAMINER SIGNATURE

Face Sheet

Name:.................................Date:............................Client Ref:..

SKIN TONES
Light
Medium
Dark

FOUNDATION & CONCEALER

SKIN ONDITIONS
Young
Mature

EYES

MAKE-UP CONTEXTS
Day
Evening
Bridal

TECHNIQUES
Correction - Warming
Correction - Cooling
Concealing
Bronzing
Highlighting
Shading
Strip Lashes
Individual Lashes

CHEEKS

FASHION STYLE

LIPS

PERIOD STYLE

ADDITIONAL TECHNIQUES

Note:

Is this client contraindicated?   ☐ YES   ☐ NO

This is evidence of:

☐ Class Work   ☐ Home Work   ☐ Internal Evaluation   ☐ External Examination

CONTRA-ACTIONS	
AFTERCARE ADVICE	
HOME CARE ADVICE	
CLIENT/ MODEL SIGNATURE	TEACHER/ EXAMINER SIGNATURE

Face Sheet

Name:............................Date:............................Client Ref:..

SKIN TONES
Light
Medium
Dark

SKIN ONDITIONS
Young
Mature

MAKE-UP CONTEXTS
Day
Evening
Bridal

TECHNIQUES
Correction - Warming
Correction - Cooling
Concealing
Bronzing
Highlighting
Shading
Strip Lashes
Individual Lashes

FASHION STYLE

PERIOD STYLE

ADDITIONAL TECHNIQUES

FOUNDATION & CONCEALER

EYES

CHEEKS

LIPS

Note:

Is this client contraindicated? ☐ YES ☐ NO

This is evidence of:

☐ Class Work ☐ Home Work ☐ Internal Evaluation ☐ External Examination

CONTRA-ACTIONS	
AFTERCARE ADVICE	
HOME CARE ADVICE	
CLIENT/ MODEL SIGNATURE	TEACHER/ EXAMINER SIGNATURE

Face Sheet

Name:.................................Date:...........................Client Ref:..

SKIN TONES	FOUNDATION & CONCEALER
Light	☐
Medium	☐
Dark	☐

SKIN ONDITIONS

Young	☐
Mature	☐

EYES

MAKE-UP CONTEXTS

Day	☐
Evening	☐
Bridal	☐

TECHNIQUES

Correction - Warming	☐
Correction - Cooling	☐
Concealing	☐
Bronzing	☐

CHEEKS

Highlighting	☐
Shading	☐
Strip Lashes	☐
Individual Lashes	☐

FASHION STYLE

LIPS

☐

PERIOD STYLE

☐

☐

ADDITIONAL TECHNIQUES

Note:

Is this client contraindicated?   ☐ YES   ☐ NO

This is evidence of:

☐ Class Work   ☐ Home Work   ☐ Internal Evaluation   ☐ External Examination

CONTRA-ACTIONS	
AFTERCARE ADVICE	
HOME CARE ADVICE	
CLIENT/ MODEL SIGNATURE	TEACHER/ EXAMINER SIGNATURE

Face Sheet

Name:................................Date:..........................Client Ref:.................................

SKIN TONES	FOUNDATION & CONCEALER
Light	☐
Medium	☐
Dark	☐

SKIN ONDITIONS

Young	☐
Mature	EYES

MAKE-UP CONTEXTS

Day	☐
Evening	☐
Bridal	☐

TECHNIQUES

Correction - Warming	☐
Correction - Cooling	☐
Concealing	☐
Bronzing	CHEEKS
Highlighting	☐
Shading	☐
Strip Lashes	☐
Individual Lashes	☐

FASHION STYLE — LIPS

☐

PERIOD STYLE

☐ ☐

ADDITIONAL TECHNIQUES

Note:

Is this client contraindicated?   ☐ YES   ☐ NO

This is evidence of:

☐ Class Work   ☐ Home Work   ☐ Internal Evaluation   ☐ External Examination

CONTRA-ACTIONS	
AFTERCARE ADVICE	
HOME CARE ADVICE	
CLIENT/ MODEL SIGNATURE	TEACHER/ EXAMINER SIGNATURE

Face Sheet

Name:..Date:..............................Client Ref:...

SKIN TONES
Light
Medium
Dark

SKIN ONDITIONS
Young
Mature

MAKE-UP CONTEXTS
Day
Evening
Bridal

TECHNIQUES
Correction - Warming
Correction - Cooling
Concealing
Bronzing
Highlighting
Shading
Strip Lashes
Individual Lashes

FASHION STYLE

PERIOD STYLE

ADDITIONAL TECHNIQUES

FOUNDATION & CONCEALER

EYES

CHEEKS

LIPS

Note:

Is this client contraindicated? ☐ YES ☐ NO

This is evidence of:

☐ Class Work ☐ Home Work ☐ Internal Evaluation ☐ External Examination

CONTRA-ACTIONS	
AFTERCARE ADVICE	
HOME CARE ADVICE	
CLIENT/ MODEL SIGNATURE	TEACHER/ EXAMINER SIGNATURE

Face Sheet

Name:........................ Date:........................ Client Ref:........................

	FOUNDATION & CONCEALER

SKIN TONES
Light ☐
Medium ☐
Dark ☐

SKIN ONDITIONS
Young ☐
Mature ☐

EYES

MAKE-UP CONTEXTS
Day ☐
Evening ☐
Bridal ☐

TECHNIQUES
Correction - Warming ☐
Correction - Cooling ☐
Concealing ☐
Bronzing ☐

CHEEKS

Highlighting ☐
Shading ☐
Strip Lashes ☐
Individual Lashes ☐

FASHION STYLE

LIPS
☐
☐

PERIOD STYLE
☐
☐

ADDITIONAL TECHNIQUES

Note:

Is this client contraindicated? ☐ YES ☐ NO

This is evidence of:

☐ Class Work ☐ Home Work ☐ Internal Evaluation ☐ External Examination

CONTRA-ACTIONS	
AFTERCARE ADVICE	
HOME CARE ADVICE	
CLIENT/ MODEL SIGNATURE	TEACHER/ EXAMINER SIGNATURE

Face Sheet

Name:.................................Date:...........................Client Ref:...

SKIN TONES	
Light	
Medium	
Dark	

SKIN ONDITIONS	
Young	
Mature	

MAKE-UP CONTEXTS	
Day	
Evening	
Bridal	

TECHNIQUES	
Correction - Warming	
Correction - Cooling	
Concealing	
Bronzing	
Highlighting	
Shading	
Strip Lashes	
Individual Lashes	

FASHION STYLE

PERIOD STYLE

ADDITIONAL TECHNIQUES

FOUNDATION & CONCEALER

EYES

CHEEKS

LIPS

Note:

Is this client contraindicated? ☐ YES ☐ NO

This is evidence of:

☐ Class Work ☐ Home Work ☐ Internal Evaluation ☐ External Examination

CONTRA-ACTIONS	
AFTERCARE ADVICE	
HOME CARE ADVICE	
CLIENT/ MODEL SIGNATURE	TEACHER/ EXAMINER SIGNATURE

Face Sheet

Name:................................Date:..............................Client Ref:...

SKIN TONES

- Light
- Medium
- Dark

SKIN ONDITIONS

- Young
- Mature

MAKE-UP CONTEXTS

- Day
- Evening
- Bridal

TECHNIQUES

- Correction - Warming
- Correction - Cooling
- Concealing
- Bronzing
- Highlighting
- Shading
- Strip Lashes
- Individual Lashes

FASHION STYLE

PERIOD STYLE

ADDITIONAL TECHNIQUES

FOUNDATION & CONCEALER

EYES

CHEEKS

LIPS

Note:

Is this client contraindicated?　☐ YES　☐ NO

This is evidence of:

☐ Class Work　☐ Home Work　☐ Internal Evaluation　☐ External Examination

CONTRA-ACTIONS	
AFTERCARE ADVICE	
HOME CARE ADVICE	
CLIENT/ MODEL SIGNATURE	TEACHER/ EXAMINER SIGNATURE

Face Sheet

Name:.....................................Date:.........................Client Ref:...

FOUNDATION & CONCEALER

SKIN TONES
- Light
- Medium
- Dark

SKIN ONDITIONS
- Young
- Mature

EYES

MAKE-UP CONTEXTS
- Day
- Evening
- Bridal

TECHNIQUES
- Correction - Warming
- Correction - Cooling
- Concealing
- Bronzing
- Highlighting
- Shading
- Strip Lashes
- Individual Lashes

CHEEKS

FASHION STYLE

LIPS

PERIOD STYLE

ADDITIONAL TECHNIQUES

Note:

Is this client contraindicated? ☐ YES ☐ NO

This is evidence of:

☐ Class Work ☐ Home Work ☐ Internal Evaluation ☐ External Examination

CONTRA-ACTIONS	
AFTERCARE ADVICE	
HOME CARE ADVICE	
CLIENT/ MODEL SIGNATURE	TEACHER/ EXAMINER SIGNATURE

Face Sheet

Name:...................................Date:...........................Client Ref:...

SKIN TONES	FOUNDATION & CONCEALER

SKIN TONES
- Light
- Medium
- Dark

SKIN ONDITIONS
- Young
- Mature

MAKE-UP CONTEXTS
- Day
- Evening
- Bridal

TECHNIQUES
- Correction - Warming
- Correction - Cooling
- Concealing
- Bronzing
- Highlighting
- Shading
- Strip Lashes
- Individual Lashes

FASHION STYLE

PERIOD STYLE

ADDITIONAL TECHNIQUES

FOUNDATION & CONCEALER

EYES

CHEEKS

LIPS

Note:

Is this client contraindicated? ☐ YES ☐ NO

This is evidence of:

☐ Class Work ☐ Home Work ☐ Internal Evaluation ☐ External Examination

CONTRA-ACTIONS	
AFTERCARE ADVICE	
HOME CARE ADVICE	
CLIENT/ MODEL SIGNATURE	TEACHER/ EXAMINER SIGNATURE

Face Sheet

Name:.................................Date:......................Client Ref:..................................

SKIN TONES
Light
Medium
Dark

SKIN ONDITIONS
Young
Mature

MAKE-UP CONTEXTS
Day
Evening
Bridal

TECHNIQUES
Correction - Warming
Correction - Cooling
Concealing
Bronzing
Highlighting
Shading
Strip Lashes
Individual Lashes

FASHION STYLE

PERIOD STYLE

ADDITIONAL TECHNIQUES

FOUNDATION & CONCEALER

EYES

CHEEKS

LIPS

Note:

Is this client contraindicated? ☐ YES ☐ NO

This is evidence of:

☐ Class Work   ☐ Home Work   ☐ Internal Evaluation   ☐ External Examination

CONTRA-ACTIONS	
AFTERCARE ADVICE	
HOME CARE ADVICE	
CLIENT/ MODEL SIGNATURE	TEACHER/ EXAMINER SIGNATURE

Face Sheet

Name:.................................Date:...........................Client Ref:...

SKIN TONES	
Light	
Medium	
Dark	

FOUNDATION & CONCEALER

SKIN ONDITIONS	
Young	
Mature	

EYES

MAKE-UP CONTEXTS	
Day	
Evening	
Bridal	

TECHNIQUES	
Correction - Warming	
Correction - Cooling	
Concealing	
Bronzing	
Highlighting	
Shading	
Strip Lashes	
Individual Lashes	

CHEEKS

FASHION STYLE

LIPS

PERIOD STYLE

ADDITIONAL TECHNIQUES

Note:

Is this client contraindicated? ☐ YES ☐ NO

This is evidence of:

☐ Class Work ☐ Home Work ☐ Internal Evaluation ☐ External Examination

CONTRA-ACTIONS	
AFTERCARE ADVICE	
HOME CARE ADVICE	
CLIENT/ MODEL SIGNATURE	TEACHER/ EXAMINER SIGNATURE

Face Sheet

Name:..............................Date:...........................Client Ref:...................................

SKIN TONES

Light

Medium

Dark

SKIN ONDITIONS

Young

Mature

MAKE-UP CONTEXTS

Day

Evening

Bridal

TECHNIQUES

Correction - Warming

Correction - Cooling

Concealing

Bronzing

Highlighting

Shading

Strip Lashes

Individual Lashes

FASHION STYLE

PERIOD STYLE

ADDITIONAL TECHNIQUES

FOUNDATION & CONCEALER

EYES

CHEEKS

LIPS

Note:

Is this client contraindicated? ☐ YES ☐ NO

This is evidence of:

☐ Class Work ☐ Home Work ☐ Internal Evaluation ☐ External Examination

CONTRA-ACTIONS	
AFTERCARE ADVICE	
HOME CARE ADVICE	
CLIENT/ MODEL SIGNATURE	TEACHER/ EXAMINER SIGNATURE

Face Sheet

Name:...................................Date:...........................Client Ref:...

SKIN TONES	FOUNDATION & CONCEALER
Light	
Medium	
Dark	

SKIN ONDITIONS

Young	
Mature	EYES

MAKE-UP CONTEXTS

Day	
Evening	
Bridal	

TECHNIQUES

Correction - Warming	
Correction - Cooling	
Concealing	
Bronzing	CHEEKS
Highlighting	
Shading	
Strip Lashes	
Individual Lashes	

FASHION STYLE — LIPS

PERIOD STYLE

ADDITIONAL TECHNIQUES

Note:

Is this client contraindicated? ☐ YES ☐ NO

This is evidence of:

☐ Class Work ☐ Home Work ☐ Internal Evaluation ☐ External Examination

CONTRA-ACTIONS	
AFTERCARE ADVICE	
HOME CARE ADVICE	
CLIENT/ MODEL SIGNATURE	TEACHER/ EXAMINER SIGNATURE

Face Sheet

Name:.................................Date:.............................Client Ref:..

FOUNDATION & CONCEALER

SKIN TONES
Light
Medium
Dark

SKIN ONDITIONS
Young
Mature

EYES

MAKE-UP CONTEXTS
Day
Evening
Bridal

TECHNIQUES
Correction - Warming
Correction - Cooling
Concealing
Bronzing
Highlighting
Shading
Strip Lashes
Individual Lashes

CHEEKS

FASHION STYLE

LIPS

PERIOD STYLE

ADDITIONAL TECHNIQUES

Note:

Is this client contraindicated? ☐ YES ☐ NO

This is evidence of:

☐ Class Work ☐ Home Work ☐ Internal Evaluation ☐ External Examination

CONTRA-ACTIONS	
AFTERCARE ADVICE	
HOME CARE ADVICE	
CLIENT/ MODEL SIGNATURE	TEACHER/ EXAMINER SIGNATURE

Are you in the mood of colouring even more?
- have a look at the rest of Julian books -

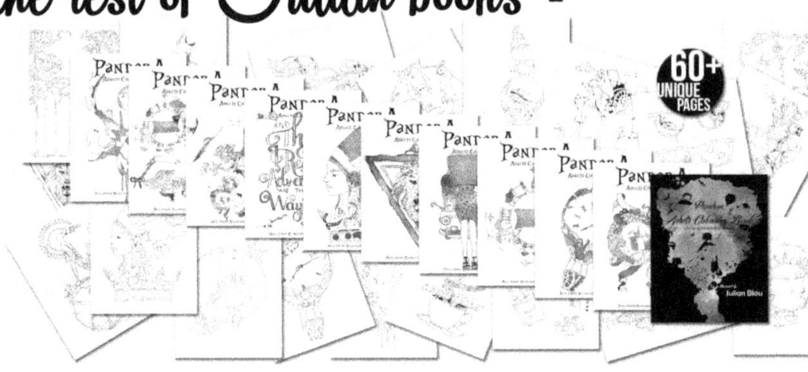

PANDORA
COLLECTION

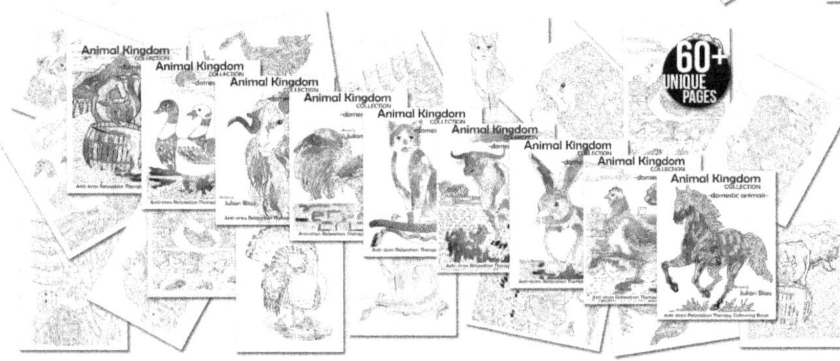

Animal Kingdom
COLLECTION

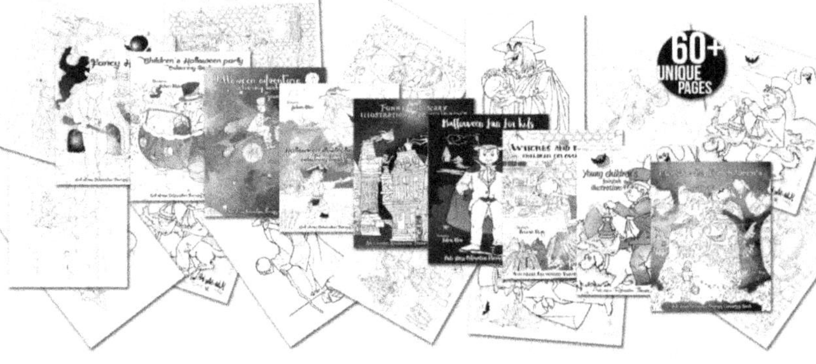

Children's Halloween
Collection

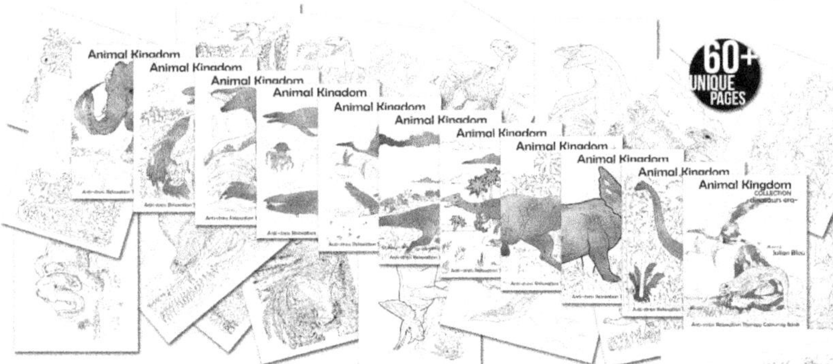

Animal Kingdom
COLLECTION
-dinosaurs era-

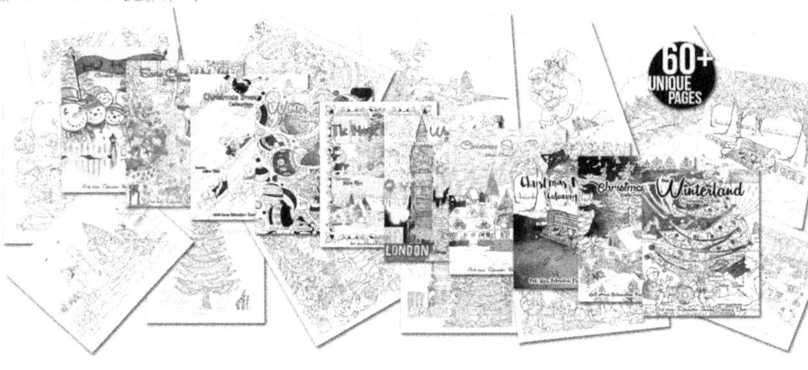

Winter Collection

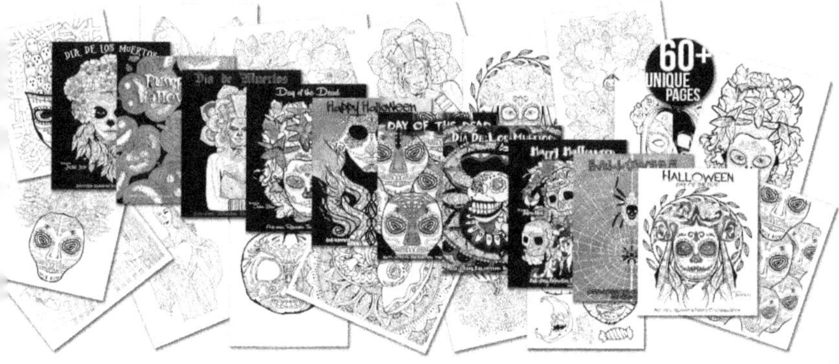

HALLOWEEN SKULLS

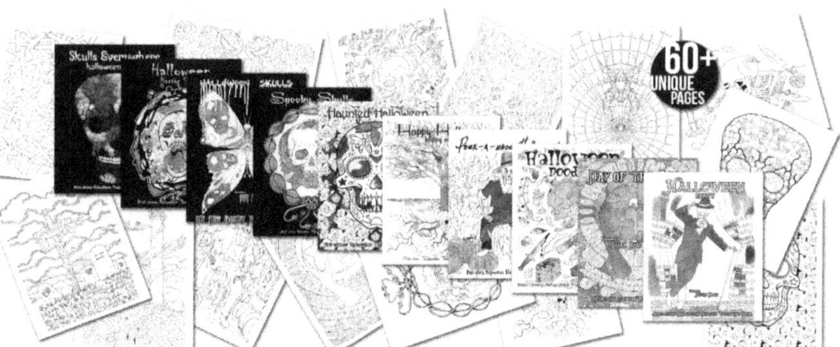

More books are added every month!

Creative Notebook Designs are coming soon :D

Face Sheet

Name:...Date:.............................Client Ref:...

SKIN TONES	FOUNDATION & CONCEALER

SKIN TONES
- Light
- Medium
- Dark

SKIN ONDITIONS
- Young
- Mature

EYES

MAKE-UP CONTEXTS
- Day
- Evening
- Bridal

TECHNIQUES
- Correction - Warming
- Correction - Cooling
- Concealing
- Bronzing
- Highlighting
- Shading
- Strip Lashes
- Individual Lashes

CHEEKS

FASHION STYLE

LIPS

PERIOD STYLE

ADDITIONAL TECHNIQUES

Note:

Is this client contraindicated? ☐ YES ☐ NO

This is evidence of:

☐ Class Work ☐ Home Work ☐ Internal Evaluation ☐ External Examination

CONTRA-ACTIONS	
AFTERCARE ADVICE	
HOME CARE ADVICE	
CLIENT/ MODEL SIGNATURE	TEACHER/ EXAMINER SIGNATURE

Thank you!